SEX
On holiday!

Levi Orion

1

AT THE CAMPFIRE!

I looked out at the sea lit by the full moon in the dark of the night.

That sounds romantic, doesn't it?

Yes, that's how it was.

A beautiful romantic night on the Spanish Mediterranean coast. It was now just after one o'clock in the morning. I've been sitting here for three hours making music. The sharp strings made my fingertips burn. The guitar was slowly getting heavy on my knees and my back was starting to hurt a bit.

But I played better than ever in my life. Not a wrong note had left my instrument tonight. No buzzing from a weakly tapped string, no discordant tone caused by a chord change in the wrong place.

I hardly understood it myself!

Actually, I don't play that well at all.

Perhaps it was the romantic atmosphere of this beach on Spain's Mediterranean coast.

I looked around and saw the real reason!

It was her!

But first things first: How did I actually end up here?

A week ago I had arrived here in Spain with my two best friends. We spend fourteen days together once a year, and have been doing so for ten years. It's already a bit of a tradition.

Every year we packed my VW bus, drove from Munich through Switzerland, France to Spain.

Somewhere we stop and rent a small cottage by the sea.

The same process every year, but always a different holiday destination. We never know where we've arrived and what we'll find. But every year it became a perfect holiday.

So also this year.

We found a small house about a hundred kilometers from Barcelona. Our daily routine consisted of beach, sea, the night program of the discotheque, alcohol and girls.

We had something else planned for tonight. We bought some bottles of red wine, some snacks and firewood in a supermarket.

Another tradition was planned tonight!

Campfire and guitar music!

I forgot to mention that I'm a musician, sing quite well and play the guitar passable.

The hours by the fire passed.

We ate, drank, laughed, drank, celebrated and drank even more. As every year, more and more strangers came to the campfire. Through the glow of the fire and my guitar music we could be heard from afar and attracted the holiday romantics like moths to a light.

Therein lay the attraction.

Complete strangers sitting together around a campfire, drinking red wine, enjoying the beach and the sea and talking.

In the meantime, more than twenty people were already sitting around our campfire. Small groups had found themselves everywhere, chatting animatedly. Everyone seemed to be having a great time.

I was completely absorbed in my musical world, so I didn't even notice that a pretty blonde girl had sat down next to me. She didn't say a word, looked dreamily at the sea and listened to my music.

During a pause she looked at me with her bright blue eyes.

"My name is Ela," she introduced herself.

"Henri," I answered only briefly, because in such a situation I always lacked the words.

"You have a beautiful voice," I heard her soft voice.

I was at a loss for words again. I wanted to say that the sparkle in her eyes is more beautiful than any tone of my voice. But of course I didn't dare and went to safe territory.

We talked about music.

Within a very short time we knew everything about each other's taste in music. I told her about my old band and shortly afterwards found out that until recently she had sung in a band herself. That she stopped there was probably related to the fact that the drummer was her new ex-boyfriend.

"May I stay with you, or am I disturbing you?" she asked me.

"If you sing something too," I replied.

She blushed slightly but nodded her head.

By now it was getting pretty dark. The air of the summer night had cooled a little. The fire bathed his surroundings in a warming light. The sparks flew into the clear night sky and mingled with the stars.

The first had already left. Some sat by the sea, others around the fireplace and watched me start another song. My voice isn't spectacular, but Ela seemed to like it.

That was the only thing that mattered to me.

I wanted to hear your voice!

And what I heard next almost left me speechless. As if it had been rehearsed a hundred times, it kicked in in the chorus. To this day I don't quite understand how such a full and strong voice can come from such a delicate being.

By now, at the latest, everyone who hadn't been drawn in by my singing was on their way to the fire to see who was singing.

I played the chorus over and over again and each time she varied the melody differently. We must have played the same part of this song for almost five minutes without anyone getting bored.

Finding more songs to play together was a breeze. We had the same taste in music and knew the same songs. One after the other we played as if we had been making music together for years.

I've never experienced campfire music silencing the audience. Normally you just add a bit of music to people's conversations. But tonight nobody dared to speak. Everyone was afraid of missing a single note of Ela's singing.

I too was captivated by her!

Her voice captivated me from the first moment. Very quietly and sparingly I accompanied her singing with my old guitar. I was almost ashamed that I had to accompany such a fantastic singer on such a shabby instrument. Everyone listened to us, even the fire seemed to dance to the beat of our music.

The people around us become fewer and fewer over time. But she still sits next to me and holds me captive with her voice.

Shortly before three o'clock in the morning we only sit alone at the campfire. We hadn't noticed how one after the other had left.

As long as we played, her gaze disappeared somewhere between the slowly diminishing flames of the fire.

My eyes were glued to her the whole time.

I watched her lips form each sound, thought I could make out each note traveling up her throat, and watched her chest rise and fall with each breath.

Then came the last note of this song.

She smiled at me. I couldn't speak a word but smiled back softly.

A loud "PLING" tore us out of our rigidity.

My D string broke!

"Looks like we've played enough for today," she said, a regretful look on her face. With a heavy heart, I put my guitar aside.

She came to me naturally, sat close to my side and put her arm around my shoulders. I enjoyed the weight of her head resting on my shoulder.

It was wonderful to feel her so close to me. Her warmth and closeness did me good. Only now did I notice how cool it had become. Without breaking away from her, I grabbed the stack of remaining firewood and added a few logs.

The blazing flames quickly drove the cold away. Nevertheless, she snuggled closer and closer to me, as if she were still freezing.

I felt her hand on my back, noticed how she pushed under the fabric of my shirt and felt her cold fingers directly on my skin.

We just sat there forever and enjoyed each other's closeness and warmth. The world around us didn't seem so important anymore. The murmur of strange voices stopped. Even the flames of the fire seemed to dance more slowly, just not to disturb the stillness of the moment. The world just stood still!

Without my noticing, we suddenly looked at each other. In the twilight her blue eyes seemed so deep I wanted to drown in them. Her features shimmered in the red and yellow of the fire. I stroked a strand of hair from her face with one finger and pushed it behind her ear. As if by itself, her cheek nestled against my palm. I slowly brought her face to mine. Only millimeters separated our lips.

The kiss drove away all the cold!

Her lips were so delicate and soft that the touch went through me to the last corner of my body. I opened my mouth a little and grazed her bottom lip with my tongue. As if waiting for that little signal, she let me in.

The kiss that started so gently became more and more passionate and demanding. She greeted me with her tongue and a wild, wet and hot dance began between our lips. Her hand was still stroking my back. I could feel her fingernails scraping the thin fabric of my shirt. The footprints they leave burned as hot as the fire next to us.

My hands also began to explore her body. With my left hand I pushed her top up a little and touched the soft skin of her flat stomach. I placed my right hand on her thigh and gently began to push her skirt up. I felt her panties with the tips of my fingers. I slowly rubbed the thin fabric that stretched over the gorgeous curves of her hips.

She looked at me in surprise as I pulled away from her and stood up. She stood in front of me immediately.

She gave me just a quick, fleeting kiss before laying down on the soft sand of the beach. Stretched out on her back, elbows propped up, she presented her body to me as if to say "come to me". A smile played around her lips. She seemed to be able to fulfill every wish and longing I had ever had.

The flickering light of the fire made her face look almost unnaturally beautiful. The entire scene seemed more like a dream than reality. The soft sand below us, the fire beside us and the stars above us.

But anyway, if it's a dream I'll enjoy it while I can and every means was fine for me now to not wake up.

Without wasting any more time or unnecessary words, I laid down next to the girl and sought her lips for another kiss. Our tongues found each other again in a passionate dance.

Very close I felt her hot, trembling body. I felt her pushing towards me. Her fingernails were on my back again. Her soft, full breast pressed against me, her abdomen pressed against me.

Surely she could already feel my excitement penetrating the fabric of my pants. With every movement of her body she rubbed against my erection. She seemed to enjoy teasing me.

With a jerk, she wrapped one leg around my waist and pulled me even closer to her. We had to break our kiss for a moment as she pressed so hard against my lap.

A common groan sounded in the night.

We lay still for a few seconds, looking straight into each other's eyes, followed by a smile and a quick movement from her. She climbed over me and sat on my abdomen.

Her face told me what she wanted.

She slowly unbuttoned her top while her pelvis continued to circle over my lap. This movement almost drove me insane. Only a few layers of fabric prevented me from penetrating her. A quick jerk of her shoulders and the blouse slid to the floor.

I leaned up and kissed her neck and the skin not covered by the skimpy bra. Her hand on the back of my head pulled me even tighter between her breasts.

That annoying piece of fabric that wanted to keep her curves from me had to go. With my greedy fingers I groped her back and undid the clasp of her bra. Nothing stood in the way of my caresses anymore. I kissed the soft skin of her plump curves and felt how every contact of my lips chased a new electric shock through her body. A soft moan escaped her lips as my tongue caressed one of her buds for the first time. Her body jerked in my arms as I gently massaged her nipples with my lips.

Now she began to undress me. With firm movements she undid the buttons of my shirt. Without being hindered by disturbing material, I now felt her fingers on my skin. She leaned down and kissed up my neck until she reached my mouth and we kissed deeply again.

Then I felt her slim body lying on me.

Her weight, her warmth, her skin.

Pure and unadulterated!

Our bodies rubbed against each other so hard, as if we wanted to be one rather than two separate people. My hands caressed her back and pulled her even closer to me.

Then I pushed her skirt up and massaged her firm buttocks. My fingers gently slipped under the fabric of her panties-

I gently worked the soft, warm skin and felt it meet my every movement.

Too much for me!

Losing all restraint, I hugged her tightly and turned her onto her back again. Groaning, she tilted her head back as I kissed her neck.

She arched her back tensely as I began massaging her breasts with both hands and my mouth kissed her nipples. It only took seconds of my tongue's play before your buds perked up.

Her hands cupped my head.

She now set the direction and speed in which my tenderness wandered over her body. Her stomach twitched with each subsequent kiss from me. I stayed on her navel for a particularly long time because she seemed very sensitive here.

Every little kiss, every tongue, every breath of air made her body shiver beneath me. She let me linger here for less time than I would have liked, before the pressure of her hands unequivocally directed me further toward the center of her pleasure. I glanced up with a mischievous grin as I unzipped the black skirt.

With impatient eyes she awaited my coming action.

I slowly began to pull her panties down. She immediately raised her pelvis slightly to help me.

Then she lay completely naked at the mercy of my eyes!

She was so beautiful!

Just a kiss on her thigh made her body tremble. My lips slowly moved up. Each of my touches was accompanied by a whimper that increased in pitch and volume.

Even the sounds of her desire sounded like music to my ears. She spread her legs slightly, gave me more space and wanted to make it easier for me to access her center.

In the firelight I saw the wet glow that already surrounded her crevices. Her scent enveloped my senses and mingled with the smell of soft grass and fire.

Her moans sounded like a song in my ear as my tongue stroked her swollen labia for the first time. I repeated these movements a few times and watched with interest how her back straightened more and more. She pushed her pelvis against me more and more wildly and her moans got louder and louder.

She was already very close to the limit of her climax.

When my lips encircled her pearl and without warning I penetrated her vagina with two fingers, only a few seconds passed before the orgasm overran her.

Waves of pleasure ran through her entire body. Her pelvic muscles rhythmically encircled my fingers as if she wanted to pull me further into her.

It seemed to take ages before her lust slowly subsided and the grip on her legs relaxed.

Without breaking the contact between my lips and her skin, I slowly licked her body back up. I let her savor the taste of her lust from my tongue.

Completely relaxed, she was now lying under me and returned my kiss while she held me weakly wrapped in her arms.

The flames next to us were almost gone, but the cold of the night couldn't harm our overheated bodies at this hour. Our bodies snuggled close together.

I slowly took off my pants. She watched everything with curious eyes. The thin fabric of my shorts was now all that stood in the way of our union.

Her breathing quickened as she studied the bulge of my panties. Then she pushed her privates firmly against my shorts and started rubbing against me.

I felt the lust in my body almost painfully. Every beat of my heart seemed to only serve to pump more blood into my bulging erect penis.

Her hands slid down my back to the waistband of my panties. She slowly pulled the fabric down on me to erase this last boundary between us.

Carefully, to savor our desire for as long as possible, I lay down on top of her. I propped myself up on my elbows so as not to put my entire weight on her and still feel her whole body against my skin.

A few times I let my glans slide down her crack. Each time I parted her labia a little further and penetrated deeper into her.

I could hardly contain my anticipation!

With a sudden movement of my pelvis I was inside her!

I felt her wet warmth enveloping me, pushing against my member.

Our joint moans were the only sound at that moment. For the second time that night, our music filled the area. None of us was interested in who was still listening to us. All that mattered was us and our feelings for each other.

For a moment we remained motionless and enjoyed the moment of our union.

Then I began to move inside her and felt her follow the rhythm of my thrusts.

Her entire body rubbed against me.

Tilting her head back, she presented her beautiful neck to me. As if by itself, my lips glided over it, covering the delicate skin with kisses.

I quickened our beat a little and could feel the tension building in every muscle of her body. She tried to spread her legs further and further to feel my penis even deeper inside her.

Her wet cave encircled me tighter and tighter.

Each movement increased our pleasure, accelerated our rhythm and brought us closer to a shared climax. Only a fine line separated us from the redeeming euphoria of orgasm. She wrapped her legs around me again and with a violent jerk she pulled me even deeper into her.

With this movement, in this moment the time had come!

The groans of our joint explosion filled the night.

Birds took flight and the fire that had long since gone out flares up for us one last time.

Every muscle was strained to the breaking point.

Every thought had left the mind to make way for this overwhelming feeling!

The moon and the stars smiled down on us. The night turned again as we lay exhausted and happy next to the remaining embers of the fire pit.

The cool air found its way into our limbs. Although everything in me was reluctant to release her from my arms, I stood up and, naked as I was, walked to my beach bag. I grabbed two blankets and rushed back to her.

As I listened into the darkness, I could hear other lovers moaning. For the second time today, our music cast a spell over our listeners. Our song together had carried our desire and lust for another loving couple.

She had meanwhile put the remaining wood on the embers and fanned the fire again.

We didn't say an unnecessary word.

The smiles on our faces told each other all that was needed. With a pleasant purr she nestled into my arms. I wrapped the blankets around us both and knew that no night, no matter how cold, could take the warmth of this moment from us.

We fell asleep next to the fire, hugging each other.

Guarded by the stars and enveloped in a wonderful night.

2

HOLIDAYS IN TURKEY!

Fly alone on vacation?

Flying alone to Turkey as a blonde, very attractive woman?

Sounds strange, but that's how it happened!

Why? I do not know it anymore.

It was August last year. My boss gave me two weeks of short-time work because there weren't enough orders over the summer months.

My girlfriends couldn't get a holiday at such short notice. I didn't have a steady boyfriend.

So what else was there for me to do?

Spend the whole day alone in Munich?

No, I didn't feel like doing that.

So I went to a travel agency and inquired about a cheap last-minute offer.

Turkey!

Only in Turkey was there a free hotel and a cheap flight.

I didn't think twice and booked the trip.

The hotel was on a beach near Antalya.

Sounded better to me than ten days in Munich.

So then: pack your bags and off to the airport.

The flight was only four hours, and the bus ride to the hotel was only an hour.

Then I finally arrived.

Alone in Turkey!

Tall, slim with long blond hair.

Apparently I caught my eye when I checked in, because I heard polyphonic whistling.

But I didn't see anyone!

Okay, it was hard to overlook me. I had selected my summer clothes before departure, a supportive bra, a t-shirt with no belly and back, denim shorts, thong and just sneakers.

At the same time, many guests had arrived, so I carried my suitcase up to the room myself. Already at 1:00 p.m. I was able to unpack my suitcase and decided to go to the beach immediately.

I changed into a baggy yellow t-shirt, black thong, black boxers and flip flops, taking my towels and sunscreen with me. I left my key at the reception and made my way to the sea.

Of course, I forgot my hotel ID, which gave me free drinks, in my room.

Never mind, I thought to myself and heard this whistle again.

This time I could make out two hotel employees!

I had to smile inwardly because both boys were at most 160 cm tall and therefore almost eight centimeters shorter than me.

But as long as they left me alone, they should whistle at me.

Arrived at the beach at this time I had a big problem getting a free lounger. I asked a hotel clerk who explained that there was a lounger for each guest. He showed me the approximate location of where mine needed to be.

After a short search I finally found the lounger with my room number.

All the seats next to me were occupied.

Then I started to cream myself. The sun in Turkey in August was very strong, so I decided to lie down in the shade.

"Shall I put lotion on your back?"

I was almost startled when a male voice sounded right next to me.

I sat up and was speechless at first.

In front of me was my dream man!

Slim, tall, muscular with short black hair.

wow!

That can't be true, I thought and swallowed.

He noticed my uncertainty and smiled.

"Did I startle you?" he asked in a gentle tone.

"No, no," I stammered in reply.

I realized I was acting like a pubescent girl meeting a boy for the first time.

I had to change that quickly because I was unsettled by his look.

I reached into my pocket and handed him my sunscreen.

"I'd love to," I said. "But only if I can put lotion on you too."

He laughed and answered in a sonorous, melodious voice.

"That's what I was going to ask for anyway."

"Okay, then I'll start," I said, getting up and standing next to him. "Lie on your stomach."

He willingly complied with my request. I knelt down next to him and slowly started creaming his muscular back.

I ran my fingers gently over his skin and felt a shiver run through his body, he seemed to be enjoying it.

Now it was my turn and I had to lie on my stomach. I threw my hair forward so my back was bare.

He paid me back!

Very, very tenderly he massaged the sunscreen into me. I enjoyed it, but he was a bit cheeky and accidentally stroked my breasts sideways, which were already noticeable.

My nipples hardened!

But he became an explorer. He stroked my spine with his fingertips, now I shivered through my body.

I hadn't recovered from that when he very carefully creamed my buttocks.

I gritted my teeth to keep from moaning!

Actually, I should have put a stop to it.

But why?

I liked it and he was the man of my previously unfulfilled dreams.

Although I thought briefly: You don't know anything about him, not even his name!

I was snapped out of these thoughts when he happily creamed my thighs, the inside of my legs.

When he then also touched the hollows of my knees particularly intensively, I had to bite my lip again to keep from groaning.

"Now that's fine," I said deliberately brash, to which he replied that he had the feeling that I had liked it very much.

Just then I looked at him and blushed!

He smiled at me and said the red suits me very well. I collected myself and thanked him.

"I'm Tobias," he then introduced himself.

"Laura," I replied.

"You only arrived today, didn't you?"

"Yes, just an hour ago."

"And right away I found you. This is my lucky day," he said, grinning.

We talked about all things God and got along great right away. Then I got thirsty.

He invited me to go to the beach bar with him. I pulled on my t-shirt and we walked to the bar. We sat close together, our knees touching.

A shiver ran through my body.

But meanwhile I didn't care either, he ordered for us and we toasted each other. We had a good chat, his fingers stroking my arm or thigh from time to time.

I felt goosebumps every time.

I could have listened to him forever, his great voice fascinated me. The time flew by. As the sun began to set, he realized it was time to go to the rooms and change for dinner.

We got the things from the couches, went into the hotel and drove up to the rooms. He lived on the same floor.

I took a long shower, then put on a slightly supportive bra, a white blouse, a black mini skirt, a white thong, and high-heeled white pumps.

So I waited and soon there was a knock.

I quickly opened the door and there he was standing in front of me.

He wore a white shirt, the top buttons undone, and smart black pants. He looked really good and smiled at me.

As we rode down the elevator, he whispered tenderly in my ear.

"You look beautiful."

We were shown to the table and had a bite to eat. I was glad when we could leave the restaurant. It was already getting dark and he asked me if we should go for a walk on the beach.

I happily agreed, as I had always imagined such a situation, walking with the man of my dreams on the beach in the moonlight under a clear starry sky.

Without asking, he took my hand. We walked slowly and wordlessly to the beach, my heart pounding in my throat.

The water rippled gently and the stars shone.

I had planned to say so much to him, I turned to him, we looked at each other and I couldn't get a sound out.

He smiled at me and nodded, as if he knew I wanted to tell him something. My throat was tight, so I just hugged him and kissed him hard on the mouth.

Now he seemed surprised.

I looked into his sparkling eyes and knew he was the one I was always looking for.

He quickly returned my kiss. Very, very tender and gentle.

The kiss seemed to last forever. When our lips parted, we walked wordlessly along the beach.

I was aroused by his nearness. The fabric of my panties was already stuck to my labia.

I wanted him!

But could I just say that?

When we reached the hotel, I grabbed his hand and pulled him to my room. I opened the door and seconds later we were in my bed.

I was lying down, he was sitting on my stomach and had pressed my hands to the right and left of my head.

"Now I'm going to torture you to death," he breathed lovingly.

"You can do anything with me," I answered, breathing quickly. "I'm yours only!"

He kissed me, nibbled my ears, tickled my neck.

Soon we were out of breath.

He undid the buttons of my blouse with one hand and played around my nipples with the fingertips of the other hand. His tongue conquered my mouth. I moaned passionately.

Now I also opened his shirt and took it off.

He kissed my breasts, took my nipples between his teeth and nibbled on them tenderly. A shiver after the other ran through my body, my fingers had meanwhile dug into his back.

Now he ripped off my miniskirt and thong with a jerk and had me naked at his disposal.

He looked at me carefully. His eyes lingered extensively on my blond triangle of pubic hair. I spread my thighs and gave him a clear view of my slit.

"You are gorgeous."

He was now full of passion!

His pants and panties landed next to the bed.

Now I asked him to lie down.

I caressed his stomach, his chest, played around his best piece and saw how his penis erected.

I carefully took his cock in my hand, pulled back his foreskin and nibbled on his glans. This did not leave him cold. He got hard and moaned.

Now I played around his glans with my tongue and jerked his shaft with my hand. Then I put it in my mouth and played around it with my tongue. I moved my head up and down, his pelvis did the same, filling my mouth completely.

Then he turned around so we could take the 69 position. He worked on my blond hairy vagina with fingers, lips and tongue. He also seemed to like my anus particularly well. Again and again he kissed and licked my sphincter.

Suddenly I felt his body begin to twitch.

His horny cock vibrated and seemed to explode!

Then he reached his climax and pumped his warm sperm down my throat. I swallowed everything and realized that his member did not lose hardness!

He was still operational.

My dream man had a dream cock!

We looked at each other laughing.

I slid forward a little and wiggled my ass invitingly.

He seemed to have understood my request and was not long in coming. I felt him straighten up and position himself behind me. His hard phallus rubbed through my wet crack.

With a single, hard push, he penetrated me completely.

I screamed my lust out loud!

I needed this now!

Without feeling and tenderness he banged me hard.

He leaned forward and twirled my hard nipples with his fingers.

I screamed with pleasure!

So at first I didn't notice how he pushed his glans through my sphincter. I wanted to turn away, squirm, but had no chance.

With a hard push he penetrated completely into my intestines!

He fucked me in the ass on our first night.

How cool was that?

My dream. Finally it comes true.

In my heart I am a submissive anal mare and I want to be taken hard.

He did it!

He fucked me so hard in my anus that I was already afraid he would tear my rosette.

After two or three thrusts, the pain gave way to boundless pleasure and I realized that I would come back soon. His cock also twitched in my intestines, but he continued to fuck me with calm thrusts for a long time.

Then the time came!

We both came at the same time, in an almost endless orgasm.

"You horny bitch," he breathed lovingly. "Lie down on your stomach."

"But I'm exhausted and I want to cuddle," I replied.

"Lie on your stomach!" he ordered more sternly.

Moisture dripped from my labia, his commanding tone made me so horny.

So I laid down on my stomach and spread my legs. Then he shoved two fingers of his left hand up my ass and started fucking me. With the other hand he massaged my clitoris.

Again I was close to an orgasm.

When he then stroked my labia and clitoris, fucked me even harder in the ass with his fingers, it was done.

What I never thought possible happened.

I got the stronger orgasm of my life.

The feelings racing through my body just wouldn't stop. I jerked all over like a fish out of water.

After I landed back on earth, we hugged and kissed. We took a shower together and lathered each other up.

I flew to Turkey alone and didn't regret it.

I can therefore recommend this beautiful holiday destination to everyone!

3

UNFAITHFUL WIFE IN BELEK!

Holiday again at last!

After the long rainy months in Munich we were looking forward to the hot sun of Turkey,

Although we had resolved never to holiday in the same place twice, we had enjoyed Belek so much last year that we booked a second time.

Oh yeah, I haven't introduced myself yet.

My name is Marcel, I'm 29 years old and unfortunately only 172 cm tall. I suffer a lot from my short height. To make matters worse, I also have a small penis. Since I don't do any sports, my figure cannot be described as attractive.

But miracles do happen in life!

I was married to an absolute dream woman. Jennifer, called Jenny for short, is very slim, has long blond hair and an immediately eye-catching bust size of 80 D. She is very proud of her appearance, especially of her hair, and takes care of herself accordingly. She is a trained tax clerk and still works in the tax office where she completed her apprenticeship.

That such a dream woman married me was a real miracle!

We live west of Munich, have been together for five years now and have been married for six months. We didn't have time for a honeymoon back then, so we made up for it in Turkey.

Turkey!

Now I knew why my wife really wanted to go to Turkey.

I now know that Jenny was friends with a Turk when she was young, who also deflowered her. She had been dating Kenan for two years and had a sexual crush on him. She did everything he wanted, trained like a puppy. To the chagrin of her parents, there was already talk of marriage. But her boyfriend at the time gave in to his family's urging and ended up marrying a Turkish girl. It happened on a so-called vacation in Turkey, just with his parents, in the village they come from. Threaded by his relatives who also chose the bride.

It was a big disappointment for Jenny and her parents were afraid she would harm herself.

I didn't know anything about that, otherwise I wouldn't have booked a holiday in Turkey.

I met Jennifer at work. The tax office where she worked also did my tax return. One day I found the courage to invite her. She accepted and married me five years later.

As I know today, she never forgot the memory of her Turkish boyfriend.

At the beginning of our relationship, I had concerns about whether I could really satisfy her with my small penis, because unfortunately it only measures twelve centimeters and is not particularly thick.

When I asked her about this physical weakness of mine, she just laughed and said that it didn't matter at all. It would just depend on how you went about it. It is important in everything that you treat each other equally and, of course, tenderly. She was fed up with the dominance and macho demeanor of her first boyfriend. Love is in the foreground in a partnership, mutual respect and trust, that you respond to your partner's wishes, take them seriously and don't treat him like an inferior person, like a slave.

I believed her every word.

It didn't matter that my penis was small.

I believed her every word.

How naive was I?

But I loved my wife, so I trusted her words. I hadn't regretted a moment of being with her in five years. In my opinion, we also had a full, satisfying sex life and were very happy together. If there were problems, we talked about them and thus hardly had any arguments.

I was sure that I satisfied my wife sufficiently.

I was really very naive!

Now we were in Turkey and had two wonderful weeks of vacation ahead of us here on the Turkish Riviera. The transfer from Antalya only took half an hour, so we arrived at the hotel around 1 p.m.

Thank god only one other couple got off the bus besides us, so there was no crowd at the reception. The room was even ready and we were able to unpack your suitcases right away.

The room was perfect. It was on the third floor in a three story wing on the left side of the complex. The balcony faced the garden with uninterrupted views over the palm trees to the sea. The weather was right, not a cloud in the blue sky, the air was 28 degrees, the sea was still a bit cold in early summer, but there was a heated pool. We met them again, all the employees of the hotel with whom we had been in close contact over the past year and they also recognized us and greeted us warmly.

Nothing should disturb our vacation!

We just wanted to relax and unwind, we just wanted to hang out and the only activities other than love, food and drink should be some exercise, lounging in the sun and short walks on the beach.

In the evening after dinner my wife wanted to go shopping. All we had to do was leave the hotel and cross the street. On the opposite side was one shop after another. There were jewellers, opticians, pharmacies, clothing stores and many more.

We knew the biggest jeans and t-shirt store from last year. We had already bought quite a few things here and had always received very good advice.

Jenny wanted to go to this store!

I didn't worry about it as I remembered the owner as being very friendly.

We rattled off various shops, but finally ended up back at Hasan's jeans and clothes shop.

This is where Jenny wanted to go!

She beamed.

How naive was I then?

The friendly Turk immediately invited us to a raki. We gratefully accepted this Turkish custom. We sat in the back of the store and within twenty minutes we had downed three rounds of raki.

How friendly the Turks are.

How naive we German husbands are!

There were two leather sofas at the back of his shop and we sat facing each other. Hasan, the 35-year-old owner, was extremely generous with his raki today. As always, he was very friendly and charming. Nevertheless, he seemed very dominant in his whole appearance, with his charisma. He is about 1.84 tall and built a bit stocky. With his dark eyes he is a real womanizer and proud of it. He describes himself as the "stallion of Belek".

After the sixth round of raki, he said to me, very confidentially, but in a way that Jenny could hear,

"Marcel, I have a hammer in my pants so big that once I fuck a woman with it, she can't get rid of my cock."

You know those sayings.

Turks usually have an exaggerated self-confidence with little background. However, he kept staring at Jenny's massive breasts. That bothered me! He literally wanted her to relate it to himself. After his words she looked at him very intensely and had a strange gleam in her eyes. Whether it was just the alcohol or the erotic content of his statement, I couldn't tell without a doubt. However, none of this aroused anger or jealousy, but rather made me, perhaps because of the slight tipsyness I was already feeling, somehow proud that my wife made such an impression on him. And again we drank a round of raki and Hasan his apple tea.

The seating area we sat on was cleverly arranged. It was probably in the shop, but was not visible from the entrance.

Now Chloé came down the stairs from Hasan's office and sat down with us. Chloé, a very attractive Swiss woman, spent her third vacation in Belek. We always met her here at

Hasan's on the three shopping trips and got to know her a little. She seemed fixated directly on Hasan.

Chloé looked beautiful with long dark brown hair and an amazing figure with a massive bust. She wore a skimpy t-shirt today that emphasized her breasts. You could tell from the bulging nipples that she wasn't wearing a bra. She also wore a tight mini skirt and high heels. The whole thing just looked hot, but had a slightly slutty touch.

First she drank a large gulp of raki from a water glass. Hasan stuck to his apple tea.

He took little notice of Chloé during our conversation, instead staring defiantly at my wife's breasts. Jenny wore a slightly transparent blouse without a bra, a thin linen jacket over it, jeans and open-toed shoes with low heels. Now that she was sitting on the couch, her jacket was slightly open so that her breasts could be seen clearly under the transparent blouse.

She showed no shame.

On the contrary!

I got the impression that she really enjoyed being able to present herself like this.

Her nipples were hard and pressed against the fabric of her blouse.

By the time we left the hotel, I had noticed that, contrary to her normal habit, she wasn't wearing a bra. But I didn't worry about that because it was very hot.

How naive can a married man be?

But as Hasan stared at my wife's barely covered breasts, I remembered that last year when we said goodbye to him, he told her that when we come back to see him, she shouldn't wear a bra anymore.

I was a little surprised that she would implement such a request, like an order!

Or was it just a coincidence?

But I couldn't and didn't want to think about it, and I didn't even have time for it because Hasan started the next attack at that moment.

Still staring at Jenny's breasts he said to me:

"You have a horny bitch! She has super udders, really great for a tit fuck. Tell her to take off her jacket and undo two more buttons on her blouse!"

Stop! Stop!

I thought and should have protested.

At least I should have gotten up and left the store with Jenny.

But what did I do?

Nothing!

Due to my now somewhat advanced alcohol consumption and also because of the hot situation, I lacked the right words.

Of course, at first I was a little shocked by Hasan's vulgar language and what he was asking of me.

My wife should undo more buttons on her blouse!

That's not possible!

Then, after a brief moment of reflection, I found it exciting. The instruction to her, which I should ask her to present herself even more here in the store, was a bit daring. But I couldn't deny the situation something tingling. Also, I didn't want to come out to Hasan as a stuffy spoilsport.

On the beach while sunbathing, she showed even more bare skin!

Now here in Hasan's shop it was probably a bit different, but the idea of seeing my Jenny sitting here with almost bare breasts made me a little horny.

I looked in Jenny's direction.

"Do what Hasan just asked for, because I too would think it would be great if we could see your tits better!"

Whether because of the vulgar way of speaking, which I had now also adopted, or because of the instruction as to what to do, she looked at me in disbelief at first. In her shiny, alcohol-marked eyes, she tolerated even less than I did, but I could also see an expression of adventure and lust.

I gave her a stern nod to emphasize the request.

She understood, first smiled at me, then at Hasan, took off her jacket and then undid the next two buttons on her blouse as requested.

The three of us watched them and Hasan said that that would be something to start with.

Jenny arched her back and thereby presented her breasts even more. You could now see the half-bare breasts, the beginning of the areolae and her hard nipples, which pushed through the fabric. The thin fabric really didn't cover the nipples and the rest of her tits.

Then there was another round of raki, in which Hasan even drank one too. Then he put his glass on the table and turned to Chloé.

"Her outfit is better that way, isn't it?"

The pretty Swiss woman examined my wife before answering dryly: "The pants are annoying! No woman with such slender legs should wear pants. That's what skirts were invented for!"

Hasan nodded.

"You're right!"

He got up and went into an adjoining room. When he returned he was holding a leather miniskirt.

He looked at me and threw me the skirt.

"Tell your blond whore to take off her pants and any pants she's wearing. Then she should put on the skirt and only the skirt, understand?"

I was outraged!

I was shocked!

The Turk called my beautiful Jenny a blonde whore!

I got hard!

Because my penis was so small, the others couldn't see the small bulge in my pants. But I could feel my hard cock rubbing against my panties.

Nevertheless, his wish went too far!

I was about to get up to put an end to it when Jenny reached over and took the miniskirt. She stood up and staggered slightly to the locker room. Now I stared at her in disbelief.

Just as she was about to close the curtain, she saw Hasan shake his head.

Leaving it open, she turned and pulled her pants down. Since she bent over, we could admire her great bare ass emphasized by the thong. To my amazement, this vulgar expression became more and more normal even in my mind.

She gave us a perky look over her shoulder and shook her butt a little. Then she stripped off her pants completely and grabbed the waistband of her panties. Slowly and erotically she pulled down the thong.

Again she wiggled her ass while bending over. Now you could even see her blond, hairy labia between her thighs.

"Look at this horny slut," Hasan said to me, licking his lips. I acknowledged it with a nod, as if it was the most natural thing in the world for my girlfriend to show off her vagina.

Completely naked from below, she turned around and presented us with her blonde bush. Then she slowly pulled up her skirt.

"Just great this blond hairy cunt. Our women all have dark brown or black pubic hair," Hasan said.

I too could not take my eyes off my wife during this performance. Forgotten was my anger at Hasan's vulgar language, I myself thought and spoke in his words.

The situation was just sharp!

I clearly noticed the bulge in my pants. Hasan noticed it too and smiled at me.

"You like it when your beautiful slut shows off really horny?" he said.

I just nodded!

I was incredibly turned on when he spoke of her in such a vulgar and dirty way.

"Yes, my wife can be a really horny slut," I heard myself say.

That is what I said?

I was beside myself now.

Jenny came back and sat down next to me, so again opposite Hasan on the couch. We then drank another round of raki.

She was about to cross her legs when Hasan shook his head again.

He looked defiantly at the hem of my wife's skirt.

"Tell your whore never to cross her legs again and also tell her to spread her legs so I can see her whore cunt better."

"You heard what to do," I said, my voice raspy.

Jenny looked me in the eyes, shifted her butt forward a bit and spread her legs. It was cool how she continued to look me in the eye and obediently carried out the order. Everyone could now see her labia lips glistening wet under the skirt that had slipped up. Even her blond pubic hair shimmered wetly.

My wife was excited!

She was so wet that her cum oozed out between her labia and ran down her legs.

"That's right!" said Hasan.

At the same moment a salesman came to the back. He addressed Hasan in Turkish.

Jenny and I were startled by this. She quickly sat up straight again, pulled her skirt right and put her left hand on the open blouse to cover her breasts a bit.

Hasan got up and went to the front with the seller. A little later he came back with a strange man. They exchanged a few words and Hasan asked him to sit down on the leather sofa. From the sound of the words, the man must be Russian. So he sat down next to Chloé, in the space Hasan had vacated, with a direct view of my wife.

Hasan stood behind him and I noticed that he was now holding a camera.

"May I introduce Jenny and Marcel and this is Chloé," pointing to each person. "This is Ivan, a good customer from Russia."

With the new guest at the table, there was a new round of raki. Glasses were filled and everyone toasted. I noticed the alcohol more and more and as I saw from Jenny's look, she felt the same or even worse. When the glasses were empty, Hasan raised his voice again.

"And now Marcel you can show us how horny it makes you when you show your slut in public like that. The bulge in your pants earlier was proof enough, now down with your pants and get your cock out. I want Jenny to see how it turns you on when she's on display."

As if under compulsion, I opened my pants, pulled them down together with my underpants and exposed my cock. Due to the interruption and the new guest, my penis had become limp and was now lying between my legs. He was so small and puny.

It made me a little nervous that Jenny, made curious by Hasan's words, was watching me

"Look, what a little tail we have there. You want to satisfy a woman like Jenny with such a tiny one?" Hasan sneered and laughed out loud. "Now bend over to your fuck bitch and open her blouse completely. Ivan will want to see what big tits your wife has."

Jenny supported herself with her hands on the couch. I opened her blouse all the way and pulled her apart. Her breasts stood out nicely, the nipples were hard and pointed 2 cm forward.

The sight and the fact that I was presenting my wife's breasts to a complete stranger excited me. My small penis swelled a little.

"Look Jenny how this turns your boyfriend on," Chloé said, pointing at my cock.

Jenny now looked at my little one with interest and registered my reawakened lust.

"And now you're going to show us all your wife's cunt! Let's go!" ordered Hasan.

As if in a trance, I bent down to Jenny again and pulled her skirt up. With a slight pressure from behind on her bottom, I asked her to slide forward again.

Then I spread her legs.

In order to give Ivan an even better insight, I pulled her outer labia apart slightly so that Ivan could really look into her wet, sputum-shining hole.

My cock was like a one.

Both Jenny and Hasan saw it.

Hasan laughed and kept taking photos of us.

At a nod from Hasan, Chloé tackled Ivan, pulled out his cock, bent over him and took it deep in her mouth.

"And now Jenny, show Ivan how to please yourself. You can also jerk off your little one," he ordered first my wife and then me.

My wife fingered her wet hole first with one, then with two and finally with three fingers. With the index finger of her other hand she massaged her clitoris wildly.

Chloé sucked smackingly and with full devotion Ivan's big cock. Jenny moaned louder and louder and I jerked harder and harder. We reached our climax together.

I squirted my semen in a high arc onto my wife's belly. Jenny had also slightly sprayed out of sheer lust. Her pleasure juice ran down her legs in small streams. The Russian poured into the mouth of the pretty Swiss woman, who had trouble swallowing the large portion.

Hasan laughed and kept snapping pictures of us.

Then Chloé got up, went to Jenny, bent over her and French kissed her. You could clearly see the tongue play of the two women. Then Chloé raised her head a bit and let her saliva and the last remnants of Ivan's sperm drip into Jenny's open mouth.

Ivan turned to Hasan.

"Can I fuck the blonde German whore?"

He pointed to my wife!

Hasan laughed and shook his head in the negative.

"The bitch isn't on sale yet, maybe next time. Today you have to make do with Chloé. But for that you can fuck her in the ass today."

Ivan got up, took Chloé's hand and took her upstairs to the office.

Too bad, I would have liked to watch the anal ascent.

"Now she's going to be properly broken in, then she'll be easier for me to take later on," said Hasan, coming around the couch and standing in front of Jenny.

"Now it's time for a blowjob, you whore," he said, grinning at me.

Jenny hesitated at first, but then opened his pants. She looked at me with a horny look and a smile on her lips and took out his penis.

I could only marvel!

Hasan really hadn't lied, his tail was a good 26 cm long and must have had a diameter of 5 cm.

What a monster!

But my wife seemed to like the sight.

I thought size didn't matter to her?

How naive was I then?

Jenny threw herself on the huge cock, like a thirst for a sip of water. She first licked the glans, then down the shaft and up again until she finally took it into her mouth.

She worked on his cock with all devotion.

She always told me she didn't like having a penis in her mouth.

Did she just mean my sex organ?

I got up, walked around the couch and stood next to the two to be able to watch the goings-on better.

I liked watching.

Was I a voyeur?

My cock was hard again.

I had just hosed down! It usually took hours for him to get stiff again.

Hasan, noticing my hard penis, pushed Jenny and pointed to my cock. She let his phallus slip out of her mouth with a pop, looked at my tiny one and laughed. Then she took

Hasan's cock back into her mouth and blew it on with all fervor.

She laughed at her husband's member while sucking a stranger's penis.

I was supposed to be enraged, instead I jerked my sweet stick.

Watching Hasan cum in my wife's mouth, pumping copious amounts of cum down her throat, I too reached my next climax.

I squirted my semen directly onto my wife's massive breasts.

Jenny submissively swallowed the foreign sperm without wasting a drop.

This, like everything else before it, was captured on camera by Hasan.

Jenny and I were still dazed when Hasan asked me to kiss her. I followed his command and French kissed her. Her mouth still clearly tasted of Hasan's sperm.

To my surprise, I didn't mind.

On the contrary!

For the first time in my life I tasted another man's sperm.

I liked it!

After that I even licked my sperm off her breasts.

Sabine's face, her tits and then also cleaned her stomach and thighs.

Hasan stands directly behind my wife.

“Your whore is really a horny slut. Can you really fuck her with your tiny one at all?” he asks me.

My mouth went all dry.

"She... uhh... she prefers it tender," I replied.

"Bullshit!"

Hasan grabbed her hips and pulled her to him.

"Your bitch wants to be fucked properly!"

I see a glint in Jenny's eyes as she felt his strap on her bare ass.

Hasan started making fucking movements, first lightly, then harder. Jenny's plump breasts bounced provocatively up and down.

"But... uhh... not really," she protests.

Hasan stopped.

"Look at your husband and tell him you don't dream of getting fucked really hard by a big cock!"

Jenny actually looked at me while Hasan rubbed her hard nipples between index finger and thumb.

"Tell him you don't want me to massage your fat udders!"

Before my eyes he massaged her big breasts roughly and hard.

Jenny moaned softly, looking me straight in the eyes.

Blood pumped into my penis again.

How was that possible?

This Turkish bastard pressed his abdomen against my wife's ass and massaged her breasts and my cock hardened.

was I a pervert?

Between her legs I saw his massive monster cock rubbing against her ass.

Jenny moaned louder and louder.

"Yes, you like that! The wimp can't offer you such a giant, can he?" he laughed arrogantly and looked at me condescendingly.

He pushed Jenny forward so that she supported herself with both arms on the back of the sofa.

Hasan stood directly behind her, tail erect.

"Come on you loser come here."

I looked at him in disbelief but moved closer so I could admire his massive penis up close.

Hansa grabbed his cock and stroked my wife's wet labia with his glans.

"Hmm... lovely wet sow," he says, grinning at me.

He grabbed her head and turned it towards me. She looked at me apologetically. I see the excitement and greed in her eyes.

He continued to rub his head against her vagina. Jenny willingly moves her abdomen.

"Look at his little one and tell him which cock you want!" Hasan challenged her.

"I...uhh...I...want your cock, Hasan. I want to feel your fat cock inside me”, she gasped and looked into my eyes.

The Turk laughed and pushed his cock slowly into her wet vagina while she moaned hornily.

Watching his giant slowly slide into my wife, I started jerking off my penis again.

"Get your hands off your cock, you loser! You can jerk off if I let you!"

Then he started fucking my wife hard from behind. He repeatedly slapped her on her buttocks.

She moaned and wailed at a volume I had never heard from her before.

Her big breasts wobbled provocatively with his hard, fast thrusts. "Oh god, is your cock awesome," my wife moaned.

It didn't take long for her first orgasm to shake her.

Hasan paused briefly and then continued to fuck hard. The Turk seemed to have sensational stamina. He fucked my wife harder and faster.

Her moans and cries of pleasure were already taking on animal features.

Hasan grabbed her long blond hair and pulled her head back.

"You like that fuck piece, don't you?" Be mounted like a bitch in heat. That's what you want, right?"

"Oh yeah... yeah... finally a great big cock. I need it so badly Give it to me, fuck me with your hot fat stud cock," she moaned.

Didn't she say size doesn't matter?

I didn't recognize her!

My small penis was so hard it hurt.

But I wasn't allowed to jerk him off, the Turk had ordered me to.

Hasan pulled his cock out of her vagina. He was glistening with moisture.

"Turn around and lie on the table, you whore!"

She immediately obeyed his command.

As soon as she was on her back, he pushed his phallus into her sex and pounded her hard and roughly.

Her big breasts rocked back and forth with every push.

"Who fucks you better? The wimp or me?" he gasped.

Jenny looked at me. The lust was reflected in her eyes.

"You... ohhh Hasan, you fuck way better than my husband. Your huge cock feels so good."

Hasan laughed out loud and continued to fuck my wife in front of my eyes. He took her from one orgasm to the next.

Her body shook as if her fingers were plugged into a socket.

Then he grabbed her, pulled her up and pushed her onto her knees in front of him.

"Open your mouth, bitch," he commanded.

He shoved his fat head into her mouth.

"You can jerk off you wimp while your wife swallows my cum," he gasped.

I had received permission to jerk off my penis.

Finally!

I felt deep gratitude.

I immediately pushed my foreskin back and forth in a rapid rhythm.

Finally jerk off!

Then I saw Hasan shaking all over. His tail twitches.

Jenny held the thick shaft covered, jerked on easily.

I recognize her frantic swallowing movements as she enjoys his cum. She never did it to me!

She told me she would never drink the male semen.

How naive was I then?

I only had to make a few jerk movements before I came again. I cum in high arcs watching my wife lick the turk's cock clean.

"You can go now," Hasan said, holding up the camera. "These are for the family album."

We got dressed with Jenny keeping on the miniskirt with no pants whatsoever. With her blouse, linen blazer and shoes, she walked to the front with me.

We said goodbye to Hassan, who pulled Jenny to himself. Outside the store, that is, publicly and in my presence, he reached under her skirt and shoved a finger into her vagina.

As he penetrated her slightly, I heard his soft voice.

"I want to fuck you again tomorrow. Get rid of your wimp."

Jenny nodded her head, pushing Hasan aside and linking my arm. Together we strolled back to our hotel.

It turned out to be an interesting holiday!

4

LISA IS ON HOLIDAY!

"I want you to come to my room with me."

Lisa couldn't believe herself that she had said those words to the young man. Her pulse was racing, a thousand thoughts shot through her head at the same time. She also couldn't believe that she had actually grabbed his hand and was now stumbling up the stairs to her room in the small hotel with him on wobbly knees.

She couldn't believe she would actually go that far. But what followed happened anyway and without her trying to regain control of the situation.

She just let it happen...

How did it come to this?

A few weeks earlier, Tobias had told her that he would not be able to take the planned vacation on the Portuguese Atlantic coast. Lisa was shocked!

Toby was vice chairman of the local football club. The first chairman, a good friend of the two, had a motorcycle accident and was injured so badly that he was now completely unable to organize and hold the big anniversary tournament to mark the club's fiftieth anniversary.

And so her husband, at first only in hints and subordinate clauses, but finally explained more and more clearly and definitely that it was a crazy idea anyway to fly on vacation so shortly before the party and only return home on the tournament weekend.

At first she had just been disappointed and sad.

The very fact that he had wanted to go away with her just before this important matter for him, she had taken that as proof that even after ten years of marriage he still loved him, that she meant more to him than his soccer buddies.

The two had married young. She was tender twenty-one when she said yes to Tobias, whom she had already met in high school.

In the years that followed, their relationship became increasingly intimate. Recently, however, her initially busy sex life had suffered a significant setback. Toby wanted to get ahead professionally, he worked a lot and was often exhausted and distracted. He had also always avoided Lisa's desire to have children on the grounds that he first wanted to "put everything in order in terms of career". And so the sex had degenerated into a rather dispassionate compulsory exercise on some weekends. Mind you, only on some!

She had told herself that was normal.

She understood, she supported him wherever she could.

She was so happy when, after some deliberation, they booked the holiday.

And now this!

In the end she had declared defiantly that she would then just go on vacation alone. And to her boundless astonishment, Toby had agreed immediately.

"Fine, darling. You relax nicely and let your legs dangle. I can then fully concentrate on the preparations for the big party. When you're back, we'll let it rip at the party."

Lisa knew exactly that having a good time meant a senseless binge with his buddies.

But she swallowed her anger, she had had more than enough of it in the last few days. So she left it at a brief "Then we're in agreement" and began to count the days until her departure.

In the days that followed, Toby didn't even notice that she was extremely disappointed and upset. He unconcernedly went back to his normal, everyday dealings with her.

When Lisa was already sitting on her packed suitcases, he had rolled on her again the night before her departure and they had mechanically fucked. Before he rolled to the side, he kissed her on the cheek and explained with a proud grin: "So you don't forget me on your vacation either."

Lisa had bitten into her pillow in the dark and didn't know whether to cry, yell or laugh.

How could he be so sure of her?

How could he be saying such things after such a lousy fuck? She lay awake for a very long time that night...

With a thick history tome, Lisa made herself comfortable on her lounger under the colorful umbrella. She was still alone on the lonely beach, which could be reached by a few steps from the hotel and which was situated in a small rocky bay.

Let's see who would show up here today.

After a week her anger hadn't dried up, but she had to think about it less and less, she quite simply forgot to be angry. She observed this in herself and knew that some things would have to change after her return. There would be a lot of long and awkward conversations. But until then she couldn't change anything anyway and so she had decided to just have a good time.

She literally came alive.

The sun, the movement in the Atlantic air, the peace and quiet and the good food in the small but fine hotel, which is a bit off the beaten path, all did her extremely well.

She had always tolerated the sun well and developed a healthy but not too deep tan. Now freckles bloomed on her nose and cleavage. This, combined with her blue eyes, gave her a youthful and perky look despite her thirty-one years. When she looked at herself in the mirror in the evening after showering, she saw an attractive woman: tall, with long legs and full breasts, firm shapes and exciting curves.

Actually made for love and overripe for having children.

She stroked her straight brown hair, which had gotten a few clear, light strands from the sun, and clicked her fingers contentedly. She hadn't felt so desirable in a long time. It's just a pity that nobody spent their vacation in this really cute hotel, with whom a little flirt would have been even remotely worthwhile.

In addition to Lisa, there was a family with a son and daughter, two elderly British couples and the small Italian women's group that Lisa classified as the "Catholic Widows'

Association Pietra Ligure". A few other guests came and went without her consciously noticing them.

She adjusted her sunglasses and continued reading, which was about the self-realization of a dishonored southern German noblewoman in the High Middle Ages.

But after just a few sentences, she was distracted again by the first approaching sun-seekers and peered over the rims of her glasses. She had always been curious and liked to observe. The happy family moved in in single file. The father with a receding hairline and a small, round tummy in front, packed like a pack donkey with everything you could possibly need for a day at the beach. Behind him his rosy wife with a flowing colorful dress and a large sun hat, also packed. The few words that Lisa had exchanged with them on various encounters had all been friendly, even heartfelt. Behind her lovely daughter, maybe 11, was doing cartwheel after cartwheel, her black braids flying around her ears. The son trotted behind him again, some distance away. So far, Lisa had only noticed him out of the corner of her eye. Possibly just eighteen, he had a book tucked under his arm. Lisa guessed that he was preparing for his high school diploma. For the first time she took a closer look at him. He tried to appear as bored as possible. Just like he doesn't belong with the rest of the group. Tall and very slim, he didn't show the slightest bit of fat. The contours of his smooth muscles showed all over his body beneath his flawless skin. His pretty little head was crowned with thick black curls, and now she also noticed his full lips, which gave his appearance something very soft despite all its harshness.

"In a few more years, then rows of women will pant after you, my little one," Lisa thought happily.

Her thoughts wandered back to her own youth, to vacations with her parents. What a stirring time. They had been in Greece when Lisa, at fifteen, was so full of hormones that she didn't know where her head was at.

Everything about her bloomed, pushed, swelled and she had to dutifully grope after her parents. How grown up she had felt when she had felt the greedy looks of Greek boys and men on her body. How much she would have liked to dance with them in the fragrant air in front of the tavern in the evening, instead she had to sit with her parents in the holiday apartment and play rummy. What a time!

She turned back to her reading.

The impoverished damsel had to fend off the impetuous advances of an unloved "cousin". But Lisa couldn't really concentrate on the story anymore. The thoughts of her own youth had stirred her up unusually and put her in a slightly tingling state of excitement. She looked up and watched as the boy got up from his towel and sauntered over to the water, deliberately nonchalant, but actually a bit awkward and uncertain. He quickened his steps, finally ran into the surf and started swimming. As she watched after him, new memories came.

Immediately after graduating from high school, she went on vacation alone with her Toby for the first time.

Her parents hadn't been overly strict with her, but they had firm ideas about what was and was not acceptable for a girl. And so Toby hadn't been allowed to stay with her until then. Sure, the two had slept together before, but the experiences were mostly hasty and not always fulfilled. In the back seat of his Golf or in a dark room at a classmate's party. So it happened that during this holiday they were able to explore and enjoy each other in peace for the first time.

The boy had meanwhile swum around one of the rocky outcrops that framed the small bay on both sides. So he had completely disappeared from Lisa's field of vision.

At that time they had only made it to the Lüneburg Heath, their longing for one another had been so intense.

With erratic movements, they had set up their small tent on the first best campsite that was on their way.

Then they had enjoyed their first freedom.

Toby was a persistent and boisterous lover with a powerful cock. The two had, with short breaks, shagged like the insane. They were evicted on the second day, as their violent games had all too obviously spilled out of the tent and the families to their right and left had complained, fearing for the salvation of their little ones. The young people then set up their tent in the open air, in a small forest, and continued to fuck. It almost came to the first upsets:

Lisa was slightly sore after days of banging. Toby felt offended when she had gently turned him away and, in his youthful impetuosity, could not sympathize with her. But a forest ranger who banished the two from the grove at that very moment gave Lisa the break she needed before the lovers could finally live out their urges elsewhere. What a time!

At some point Lisa also felt the need to cool off in the floods. She swam out, going in the same direction as the boy. With long, powerful strokes, she cut through the cold waters of the Atlantic.

She felt fresh and free. So far she hadn't swum out of sight of the hotel's beach. She was delighted to find that other bays stretched along the coast, becoming smaller, lonelier and more romantic as the distance from the hotel increased.

She decided to swim ashore behind the nearest outcrop to enjoy the peace and solitude here for a while.

This, or maybe the next bay? she thought and couldn't decide. When she finally turned inland, the hotel beach was a good distance away. You should be able to find a place to warm up here. As she got closer, the water here was just above her waist. Half walking, half swimming, she made her way between some rocks towards the beach.

Then suddenly she saw him!

Hidden from the eyes of the other vacationers, but not ten meters from her, he was standing on the beach. He leaned his back against a rock in the light surf that only lapped his ankles. His wet body glistened in the midday sun, which was high in its zenith and bathed the whole scene in a harsh white light. The spray created an almost luminous fine mist.

She now clearly saw why the boy had sought out this secluded little cove. His left hand pushed down the waistband of his swimming shorts, in his right hand he held the most beautiful cock Lisa had ever seen.

The boy's member was large and hard. Smooth and shiny, it rose steeply, streaked with fine veins, crowned by a dark, perfectly plum-shaped glans. His bulging testicles had settled very tightly against this magnificent mast.

She hadn't expected this sight!

With a short, startled whoop, she drew back.

Did the boy notice her?

Hope the sun blinded him! Instinctively she ducked into the water. Apparently the boy had taken no notice of her, for undeterred he went on with what he had started.

Lisa watched spellbound as the boy gasped and abused his club. Hissing heavily, he breathed through his closed teeth. The skin tightened over his muscles, the tendons and veins in his neck and arm bulging. His face was twisted with pain. His fist pushed back and forth over this magnificent beating, from which Lisa could no longer take her eyes off.

On the one hand she was constantly tempted to withdraw as quickly and as inconspicuously as possible so as not to get into an embarrassing situation. On the other hand, she succumbed to the fascination of the idea of doing something forbidden or even slightly shady. A feeling she hadn't felt in a long time. And finally, she was simply captivated by the sight of the enormous billet that the boy was so devotedly polishing. His movements became more erratic now, his whole body jerking slightly back and forth and his balls bobbing up and down.

Something inside Lisa told her it wasn't okay to keep watching the boy. Or maybe she was just afraid that once he came, he would notice her. Slowly and quietly, she backed her way around the crag. When she was sure that the boy would not see her anymore, she began to swim back to the hotel beach in steady strokes.

Reaching her lounger, she dried off and stretched out in the sun to warm up. But she couldn't get the image of the masturbating boy out of her mind. After a while she sat up to continue reading. The boy had meanwhile returned to his family. As if nothing had happened, he helped his younger sister build a sandcastle. As hard as Lisa tried, she couldn't manage more than two lines before she had to look over the top of her book at him again. She was fascinated by what was hidden in his swim shorts. It wasn't half an hour before the boy sauntered back towards the water, waded in and out of sight as before. As much as Lisa would have liked to know if he would do it again, she would not secretly watch him a second time.

In the course of the afternoon he made several more such "swimming excursions", as Lisa was impressed to find out. And the spectacle repeated itself several times over the following days. Lisa was delighted that she was sharing this "little" secret with the boy, while the bathing activities on the beach went on so carefree. And although her thoughts wandered to his impressive cock and toned body when she laid her hand on himself in the airy sheets of her hotel bed at night, it would not have occurred to her at that point to approach him in any way.

Too bad, Lisa thought as she watched from her breakfast table as the family boarded the coach for a two-day trip to Lisbon. She herself would start the journey home the next afternoon and so she wouldn't be able to see the boy with the big cock anymore. D

then she chuckled to herself, my condolences again. Two days of city sightseeing with mum and dad, you won't have that much time for your nice toys.

She was all the more astonished when shortly afterwards she strolled across the terrace towards the hotel beach with her bathing basket and found the boy right there with his books having a coffee.

Did she look correctly?

Wasn't he on board?

Slowly it dawned on her: he had probably gotten his parents to take this break and they had started the city trip without him so that he could study in peace.

Without further ado, Lisa changed her plan and sat two tables down to order a coffee as well. Just as she raised the steaming cup to her lips, the boy took a sip of his coffee.

Their eyes met, she smiled at him and he smiled back furtively.

My god, what am I doing here? she asked herself instantly. I'm flirting with a boy here who could be my son. Lisa, pull yourself together and take a dip in the cool Atlantic!

But she didn't do that.

Under the pretense of adjusting her chair to the sun, she turned so that the boy could admire her in all her glory. She crossed her long brown legs and continued to sip her coffee with relish. As if by accident, she tugged at her bikini top and gently stroked her heaving breasts. She was pleased to find that she found herself more attractive than she had in a long time and that the boy was glancing over at her more and more often.

What devil was she riding?

She slowly put the sweet biscuit that went with the coffee into her mouth as the Italian widows' group approached and, amid Mediterranean chatter, claimed the table between her and the boy. She landed hard in reality, grabbed her bathing suit, got up and walked to the beach.

He didn't show up here all day long.

In the evening he sat at the hotel bar with his obligatory book. Lisa had put on her favorite one-piece, light gray silk dress for the last evening, which played around her figure perfectly in all its simplicity and brought out her full breasts wonderfully. She wanted to show herself to him one last time, wanted to feel a furtive, lustful look from him one last time. If she had seriously thought about it, she probably would have sniffed herself. But the twinkle in his eyes that she had noticed on the terrace that morning had done her so much good. Unfortunately, he didn't notice this because his back was to the room and he was engrossed in his tome on a bar stool. She sat down in an armchair and leafed through a Portuguese women's magazine, lost in thought. And although she tried her best to banish the sight of the naked boy in the midday sun and the implied flirtation on the hotel terrace from her memory, the images kept coming back to her. Two martinis came to their table one after the other. For two martinis she was angry with herself. She didn't know what to do with herself and the evening that had begun. Her indecisiveness only made her more helpless.

But what should she decide to do anyway?

What was she doing here anyway?

She felt like a stupid chicken. Finally she dismissed the thought, which she hadn't really thought of yet, got up and wanted to go out onto the terrace. She walked past him, turning on her heel. She spoke to him without plan or intention.

She couldn't recall later what exactly they had talked about. It had been, quite simply, the most honest conversation she'd had in a long time.

She only remembered one thing for sure: she had not complained to him about her suffering and had not told him how she had come to this involuntary single vacation. A little surprised at first, he spoke openly and without hesitation about himself. She never would have expected that. His easy conversational style contrasted sharply with his shy demeanor when flirting on the terrace, which made him all the more attractive to Lisa. Her guess had turned out to be correct: he was actually about to graduate from high school. Without any pubertal posturing, he chatted about his plans and about the vacation.

Lisa felt her heart beat faster, her legs go weak.

She was in love.

Amorous?

That just could not be the case!

She had only known the boy for a few minutes.

The rest of the evening flew by. The bar was sparsely populated anyway and they had been the only patrons for a while. The lights were slowly dimmed to inform the last visitors that the bar was about to close.

Lisa cleared her throat, slightly embarrassed.

"Well, I'd be very happy if you might..."

She stopped. Actually, this should have been a somewhat stiff farewell. For a little eternity, neither of them said anything. And then it seemed to her that she heard herself from far away as she gently placed her hand on his thigh and said softly:

"I want you to come to my room with me."

The steps of the staircase flew towards her as if in a dream.

No sooner had the door slammed shut than he was still in the small corridor that led to the moonlit room, when he was all over her, she all over him. He smelled so wonderfully of sun and youth, he tasted so wonderfully of beach and sea. It was no longer clear who was seducing whom, even though Lisa might have shown a little more initiative at that moment.

His hands wandered up and down her body and she gasped as he squeezed her bottom and breasts through the thin silk. She made it easy for him, only a few moments later her light dress had already fallen to the ground.

His probing hands on her bare skin aroused her even more, she parted her lips. Almost greedily, as if she wanted to drink it up, her tongue went down his throat, her hands wrapped around his neck and his hard buttocks.

Finally she hastily unbuttoned his shirt and felt the warm soft skin underneath, feeling down from his chest to his hard abdominal muscles where a black fuzz trailed up to his navel.

Almost every woman would have ecstatic at this sight!

Blood pounding in her ears, she finally turned her attention to what she had already felt and sensed in her mind. She unbuttoned his pants and, without hesitation, yanked them and panties down to his ankles, kneeling in front of him as he leaned against the wall.

Then he literally jumped towards her!

He towered up and in the semidarkness of the room he seemed even bigger than she had remembered from the secret encounter in the blazing midday sun. Full of excitement and yet reverently and gently she took hold of the shaft. He was overwhelming, so hard and yet so velvety soft, she could feel his pounding pulse.

The boy groaned loudly.

Everything spun around her, she bathed in rapture that he wanted her, that he was reaching out to her, that he was stretched to the point of bursting and pushing and twitching, and a few small tears of emotion welled in her eyes .

She squeezed him tighter, gently enclosing his heavy testicles with her left hand and he moaned loudly again. Her lips approached the glistening glans.

Unbelievable, even his cock smells tempting, she thought briefly. When she finally ran the tip of her tongue along the underside, only to push her lips over the twitching fruit in one bold motion, the boy whimpered as if someone were putting the thumbscrews on him, his knees shaking.

Lisa said the pulsing of his tip was getting stronger, she wanted to give him time and pulled back, but she already felt a gush of hot liquid in her face. She kept backing away, but the next one followed, then on her neck, then another, the next landed on her breasts, another, it wouldn't stop.

The boy sank to the floor, breathing slowly and heavily.

Lisa knelt by him as he coyly stammered something about "sorry".

"No, why is that?" she answered him quickly, not wanting to

discourage him. "You're just showing how much you want me, that flatters me."

She could feel him relax a little. In the semi-darkness she gave him her happiest smile, stroked mischievously over her breasts glistening with his sauce, picked up the sticky liquid with her fingers and then licked it off with relish. She looked him straight in the eyes

"Hmm, you really are a phenomenon, the purest yummy!"

That didn't fail to have an effect, as his eyes lit up and a hint of a smile crossed his face.

"Come on, I want more of you," she said, grabbing his hands to pull him toward the bed. They stumbled into the room, and he hastily stripped off his shirt and pants around his ankles for good There was not the slightest doubt that the club, which was swinging in front of his loins and had long been straightened up again, would get even more.

Lisa took his juice from her breasts again to rub it into her slit. She wanted to be prepared for his big one. She was so excited that she hadn't even noticed that her juices had been flowing freely for a long time.

As they flopped onto the bed, he was quickly on top of her. He lay down impetuously on her and she noticed that he was heavier and stronger than he appeared in his slender build. Despite its steeply pushing size, it initially missed the entrance and she felt his hammer hot on her stomach. She gently pushed him back a little, finally grabbed him between the legs and finally directed him to her entrance. She groaned softly as he entered her in a single but infinitely slow and steady thrust.

Her breath caught for a moment!

How infinitely good that felt!

How she had waited for this!

Whether it was actually his cock or just the thought of its sheer size didn't matter to her at that moment. She was filled with him, with the weight of his body on her, with his smell and his taste. Slowly and uncertainly he began to move on top of her.

Lisa was in seventh heaven.

With Toby she had learned a few tricks over the years in order to get her money's worth when he was getting more and more callous.

She could forget all that now!

She was just horny. The gorgeous boy on top of her and his hard, gorgeous cock inside her only made her hornier and hornier. After a while, the boy's movements became more confident and bold. His excitement increased, growling softly and panting, his thrusts became more violent.

My God, how much I needed this, thought Anna.

Wordlessly, she cheered him on in her mind:

Fuck me, my big one! Give me a good thrashing! You need it, just as much as I do!

And that's exactly what he did. His rush became wilder and he drove his pelvis towards hers more and more violently. She wrapped her legs tightly around his marble ass. His powerful thrusts, with which he literally drove her across the bed, his weight on her, his hot soft skin on her stomach, her breasts, her neck and his trunk constantly jerking back and forth inside her, made her soon came to orgasm. Very hard, very intense, very strong, so much that she moaned from the depths of her throat. Her body vibrated through and through.

The boy also began to pant loudly and pushed her so vehemently as if he wanted to split her in two. Lisa tried to collect herself as far as that was possible under the circumstances. She wanted to help him, wanted to grab his balls to squeeze them, but she couldn't. Then he suddenly stopped.

Lisa felt his twitching mast in her furrow, which pulsated again.

They lay like that for a while without moving even the slightest bit. Then he slowly slid out of her and rolled to the side.

She turned to him and wanted to say something, anything. But everything that came to her mind seemed too banal and irrelevant. She had just done it with a boy who could very well have been her son. A thousand and one thoughts shot through her head.

There was only one thing she didn't have: a bad conscience towards Toby.

She had cheated on her husband and she didn't give a damn!

She was completely absorbed in the here and now. Lying on his back, he crossed his arms behind his head. His pride could not be overlooked, he literally beamed in the semidarkness. But this pride didn't seem pretentious at all, just sweet.

With a blissful smile she caressed his chest and stomach and found that his cock was still erect after the second time.

Youth is beautiful!

You have to celebrate the festivals as they come, she thought to herself, rolled on him and literally put herself on his thick rod.

Another hearty sigh sounded.

She felt as if she was going to take him in even deeper than before, as if he were running hot and softly through her gut and down her throat. She rested her hands on his chest and let her pelvis rotate slowly. She really enjoyed this position.

She soon forgot how ecstatic she had just arrived. Back and forth, up and down, back and forth she spun her bottom and almost heard the angels singing again, she was so aroused by this game. The boy gently stroked her back.

Toby had never liked that position, probably because it meant giving up too much control. It had unsettled him not to be able to determine the direction of the march. Or perhaps he was afraid of hurting himself when his tall, gorgeous wife rode him. Then it softened a few times and slipped out of her, she got a few angry looks and from then on this position was deleted from her repertoire without replacement, like so many others.

At the moment, with the boy, who was acting more and more confidently, with the Wunderhorn under her, there was no question of that at all. It rocked back and forth on its post as if tethered to it. Now she bent down to his hot lips, now she threw her head back. She shivered from tiptoe to nipple as she felt his delicious cock inside her, directing it exactly how it felt best with sleepwalking certainty. When he finally embraced her swelling breasts and gently pinched the nipples, it was over to her.

Unlike the previous one, this orgasm slowly surged in, ebbing back a little only to return more intensely. Softly whimpering, she experienced shivers after shivers and just when she thought it was over, she shook again. She had never felt anything like this in her entire life.

When it finally ended, she noticed that the boy was looking at her expectantly as she sat on him and didn't move anymore. Obviously he hadn't come, but he was still hungry. A sweet languor took possession of all her limbs. She felt a slight, not uncomfortable tug in her vagina. She knew instinctively that after this Mount Everest she would not come again. She lifted her pelvis to free herself from him, crawled to the side and stretched her butt towards him. Should he let off steam a little more on her.

At first he didn't quite understand what she wanted from him, but then he knelt behind her and willingly let her lead him. Again she grabbed his cock through her legs.

How could he still be so rock hard?

Again she led him gently but firmly to her slit to take him in at once.

She couldn't fully remember what happened next. She'd planned to squeeze the last bit of juice out of the boy's balls with a short, blustery ride from behind.

But it didn't turn out quite the way she had imagined!

He grabbed her hips and pushed her hard again. She clawed her hands into the bedding and tried to return his thrusts with equal intensity.

She wanted to finish him off, her teenage stallion!

But as if he knew exactly that, he now grabbed her tighter and took the initiative.

How he swayed his hips!

How he varied the tempo!

How he suddenly stopped, slowly withdrawing almost all the way, slowly driving back into her in full glory, only to withdraw a moment later to her gate, only to thrust again, then build up again, driving back and forth strongly and impetuously!

What a tremendous natural talent!

What a gifted fucker!

Like two great beasts mating with a thunder, their bodies smashed together on the big bed. Lisa whimpered softly and had long felt that this wouldn't be over as quickly as she had imagined...

He kept whipping her in front of him. She had long since ceased all resistance and resigned herself to her fate as his devoted mare. Any thought of humiliation was completely alien to her. She enjoyed to the fullest being coveted so much, being taken so stormily by a pretty boy full of youthful vigour. The mildest late summer night imaginable blew in from the open balcony door. Their sweaty bodies shimmered in the moonlight as they squirmed together on the large hotel bed. The crickets chirping loudly outside ensured that the gasps and moans from the room did not reach unintended ears. And again and again he gave her his sturdy scepter, and again and again she gratefully accepted the gift.

Later she didn't remember how long it had gone on like this. She hadn't noticed that whenever he pushed himself deep into her one last time, discharged himself roaring a third time, because at some point her senses had failed her.

When she awoke it was dawn. She had slept so deeply and soundly that her head was pounding slightly. She slowly realized that she had been screwed until she passed out. Her limbs were still soft as pudding.

The boy lay next to her.

For a while she looked at his slim body. His member now lay limp and heavy, but still beautiful, on his thigh. Finally she inhaled his scent one last time as she kissed his forehead gently and woke him up with a slap on his chest.

"I'm sorry, big boy, but I think it's better you go back to your room before the hotel business wakes up. It's probably in neither your interest nor mine for anyone to notice where you spent the night."

Still drowsy, he got up and got dressed, even though Lisa didn't want to take her eyes off him. Hesitantly, he finally approached her and wanted to say something, but she quickly put her finger on his lips.

"It was the most wonderful night of my life. Thank you," was all she said to him before gently but firmly pushing him out, which he let happen to him without resistance.

After gently closing the door, she took a deep breath. For the first time since yesterday, her eyes fell on the almost completely packed suitcase in the bathroom. She would arrange it so that she wouldn't run into the boy when she went to the front desk to settle the bill and have a taxi called to the airport. She had no last name, no address, nothing from him. But that didn't make her sad. It was better that way. She thought resolutely of her return to Germany.

Oh yes, things would have to change at home!

5

SKIING IN SÖLDEN!

The three of us actually wanted to go to Sölden in the Ötztal for a well-deserved winter holiday. Actually!

But then Marco called. He had suffered a capsule rupture while playing sports. He couldn't ride. But because of the costs, that's not a problem, he has travel cancellation insurance. We should drive calmly.

A week later Tim called. His boss had an assignment for him.

Sales deal in Stockholm. He didn't want to miss the chance for advancement. The boss would also bear the costs for the canceled vacation.

Great, now I had two people who paid for the holiday, but are I traveling alone? I had been looking forward to a week of skiing for a long time. But alone?

Wouldn't that get boring?

Driving down the mountains alone was only half as much fun as in a group. Sitting alone with the cyclist in the hut didn't exactly promise the desired fun factor either. But I didn't want to spend my well-earned vacation alone at home.

I was also very happy to go skiing again.

Therefore, after much deliberation, I decided to spend the holiday alone.

Due to the absence of my two friends, I had a large three-bedroom, two-bathroom apartment to myself.

I left very early on Saturday. Sölden was about two hundred kilometers away from Munich. Due to the heavy traffic on the A8 motorway, it takes me just over three hours to cover the distance.

But I reached my holiday apartment just before noon, so that I could go skiing in the afternoon.

I had left my suitcase in the apartment, I would unpack later. Just get on the slopes!

The sun was shining, the sky was blue, the slopes were pretty empty on Saturday, so almost everything was ideal. However, the snow wasn't that good. It hadn't snowed for a long time. Although the pistes were well prepared, ice sheets could form here and there.

After I got used to the feeling of having boards under my feet again, it happened. As I got braver, I slipped on a slab of ice and slid down the slope at full speed. I slid quite a bit before I was able to pivot so my feet were pointing downhill and I could press the skis into the snow to slow down.

But it was almost too late!

I slid towards a group of three people.

If that goes well.

But I was lucky.

I hit the shoe of the woman who was at the top of the group with my ski. But not so hard that she fell. She looked around in amazement, since she hadn't noticed anything about my fall beforehand.

"But be careful," she snapped at me as she pointed her skis down the valley and sped down. All I saw was white ski pants, a black jacket and long red hair that fluttered out from under the ski helmet.

Great!

Good start to the holiday. Found nice friends right away.

Dumb goat!

I got up, brushed the snow off my clothes and drove on calmly. Later I saw the group again. There were two women and a man.

I stood there for the rest of the day. No more fall. And it was a lot of fun, even if I had to drive alone.

In the afternoon I did the valley descent. Once at the bottom, I shouldered my skis to go across the parking lot to the ski bus.

Suddenly a car reversed straight towards me.

Apparently the driver didn't see me!

I slammed my hand on the trunk lid, but the car still hit my leg. Only slightly, though, before startled braking stalled it.

The door flew open.

Lo and behold, the skier with the red hair got out.

"Sorry. I haven't seen you. Has anything happened to you?"

"No. Just went well. There might be a bruise, but no problem."

"I'm sorry for that. I'm probably a bit upset. I'll give you my address. If there is anything else, you can get in touch. Of course I'll pay for everything."

Now I had the opportunity to look at them a little more intensely. The red hair suited her well. The face was narrow, with bright green eyes that could certainly sparkle when she laughed. Which of course she wasn't doing at the moment. The figure could only be guessed at under the thick ski gear, but it seemed slim and graceful. Estimated height almost 170 cm. She must be around 40 years old and her name was Natalie, as I found out from the note with the address. She lived in Nuremberg, not that far from Munich.

A Franconian!

OK, that explained a lot.

Unfortunately, Franconia is part of Bavaria, but I think it's only tolerated out of pity, because otherwise they wouldn't be accepted by any other federal state. Yes, we Upper Bavarians had a big heart.

The pretty Franconian gave me a short, sublime nod, turned around and disappeared back into her car.

I had to hurry as the ski bus was already approaching.

When I got to the apartment, I jumped under a warm shower. Then I unpacked my suitcase.

It was quite lonely, alone in a large apartment.

In the evening I walked through Sölden and looked for a good restaurant. It was a rustic hut with good food and a very good wine selection. I decided to treat myself to a bottle of red wine. Even if one bottle was a bit much for me alone. But it was my first day of vacation, so I allowed myself that luxury.

After the meal a need arose and I went to the toilet.

And who did I see on the way there?

For the third time today the red-haired Franconian!

She was sitting alone at a small table and looked glumly into a glass of coke that she had in front of her.

"Hi. So we meet again", I spoke to her friendly.

She looked up and regarded me with confused eyes.

"Uhhh... today at the parking lot. You were kind enough to snap at me," I continued.

"Oh yes," she replied. "Sorry, I didn't recognize you."

"Where are your friends?"

"Oh, that asshole," she said spontaneously. A tear rolled out of her eye.

The "A" word seemed odd coming from a beautiful woman's delicate mouth, but she must have her reason for it.

"So bad?"

"Even worse," she replied.

"Would you like to come to the table with me? I'm single too, so you can talk your frustration off if you want."

She thought for a moment and then nodded.

"I'll be gone for a moment. Then I'll come back and we can go over there."

Said and done. When I came from the toilet, she got up and pulled out from under the table a rather large duffel bag that I hadn't seen before.

Who goes to a restaurant with a holdall?

There seemed to be a bigger problem. She followed me and we sat down at my table.

"A glass of wine too? The bottle is too much for me anyway."

She agreed and quickly the waiter brought another glass.

We toasted each other.

"I'm Lukas," I offered her the "Du".

"Natalie," she answered shortly and nodded her head.

"Then tell me. What's the matter?"

“You probably saw that there were three of us on the slope. My friend Tim and my girlfriend Alina.”

I nodded my head.

"On the drive home, Tim said he had a headache and was going down. Mira joined him because she didn't have any friends skiing anyway. Because of the sunny weather, I decided to continue on my own. So we split up and wanted to meet at the hotel at five," she said in a calm voice.

She picked up her glass of red wine and took a long sip.

“I then drove for a while, but it's not that much fun alone. So I drove back to the hotel around three o'clock. Tim wasn't in our room though, although I thought he was lying down because of the headache. So I went to the balcony to smoke a cigarette. Then I hear very clear noises from the next room where Alina lives. I leaned over the parapet to see what's going on. She hadn't drawn the curtains. And there I see my Tim naked on the bed, how he fucks Alina from behind. The asshole. That bitch! We were only together three months. And then he cheats on me with my best friend! Wrong, ex-girlfriend. That stupid cow."

When Natalie tells this, tears run down her cheeks.

"I went over there, banged on the door and yelled at half the hotel. Tim opened the door naked. So I slapped him and went back to our room, threw some clothes in the holdall and ran off. I've been sitting here ever since."

"Nice crap. And now? Where are you going?"

"No idea. I asked three hotels if they still had a room. I don't want to go back to my hotel. But it's all covered."

"I can understand that you don't want to go back to your hotel. But you have to sleep somewhere. You can't sleep in the car at this temperature."

"No, of course not. I'll probably leave afterwards and drive home in my car. It's only a five-hour drive to Nuremberg."

"But that's not a good idea. In your condition on the Autobahn. Besides, you've already been drinking."

I thought for a moment.

"If you want, you can sleep in my apartment. I have enough space."

Then I told her about my friends and my unplanned solo vacation.

She agreed, somewhat suspiciously. She probably thought that I wanted to take advantage of the situation and land myself such a nice ski bunny. But that was far from my mind.

So she agreed, probably out of necessity.

We quietly finished the bottle of wine and chatted about many things, but we avoided the subject of friends very well. Then we left. I took her bag and in a few minutes we had arrived at my apartment. Upstairs I showed her the rooms and let her choose which one to take.

Then I left her alone so that she could unpack her bag.

"The bathroom is here," I then showed her the premises. To get to the bathroom, she had to go through the living room. I had chosen the room with the attached bathroom, so she had the other bathroom to herself.

Now I finally had the opportunity to take a closer look at them. As I suspected, she was slim but not too skinny. Long legs tucked into tight jeans. A firm butt. Slim stomach and a breast that wasn't too big but suited her figure. All in all, by Franconian standards, a very good-looking woman. I was amazed and impressed at the same time.

Since we were both tired, I said goodbye and wished her good night, noting that she shouldn't take it so hard.

The next morning the sun shone through the window and I got up to make breakfast. But I was late. When I entered the living room, breakfast was already on the table and Natalie was sitting behind a large, steaming cup of coffee. Slumped a bit, but apparently she was feeling a little better. However, she had teary-eyed eyes.

"Good morning," she greeted me kindly.

"Did you sleep well?"

"It was okay. Thanks."

At breakfast we talked about their plans. She didn't want to be a burden to me and wanted to drive home later today. Glad to have some entertainment, I was able to persuade her to stay a few more days. She should take advantage of the nice weather and go skiing a little. She was so looking forward to that.

After some hesitation, she agreed.

We spent a wonderful day on the slopes. Natalie seemed cheerful and happy. She was a really good skier, for a Franconian.

In the afternoon we finished at four o'clock and drove into the valley.

Freshen up at home and have a coffee. That's how you could enjoy life. Natalie had loosened up more and more throughout the day. But now something was bothering her.

"What's happening?"

"I didn't pack all of my stuff yesterday when I ran off like that.

Only the essentials. Would you go to the hotel with me to get the rest? I'm scared of facing Tim alone."

"Sure, we can do it. It's best if we leave right away, then you'll have it behind you."

When we got to the hotel, we went straight to her room. She knocked and a short time later Tim opened the door.

"Do not say a word. I just want to get my clothes. Then I'm gone again."

"Oh no. Make such a fuss yesterday and find a new lover today," he said cockily in his whispering Franconian dialect.

No, that is not possible at all!

I approached him.

"Calm down, little one," I whispered with a dangerous undertone.

He withdrew and sat down in a chair, very well behaved and intimidated. Stop Frank!

Natalie packed up her things and in five minutes we were gone.

"Thanks. I would never have done it alone. I probably would have given up my things. And all because of that stupid arse..."

"Stop," I interrupted her. "Not always that word. He's not worth getting upset about either. Even if it still hurts, forget him as soon as possible!"

"I'll try it. I just want to go skiing for a few more days if I'm not too much of a bother to you," she winked at me.

"I'm glad when I have someone to talk to. Vacation all alone is a bit dull."

The next day was bright sunshine again. It was fun driving with her. I had a much higher level, but she made up for it with cheek and courage.

In the evening we went out to eat again and everyone went to bed.

It continued like this on Tuesday.

The sun was shining and we drove the right routes again. In the evening after the shower I sat in the living room and read the newspaper.

Apparently Natalie wasn't finished yet. After ten minutes the bathroom door opened and she came out. She wore black lace panties with a matching bra.

My jaw nearly dropped.

She just looked sensational. Her body had a perfection that reminded me of a Greek goddess.

"Excuse me. I thought you weren't done yet. I'll get dressed."

I was about to tell her not to wear anything else from now on, but she quickly disappeared into her room, giving me one last look at her amazing butt.

What was that butt!

She had a tight, toned bottom that moved gracefully as she walked. My penis liked this too, because it began to erect, beaming with joy.

When she came back in a fluffy tracksuit, I kept thinking about what she was wearing underneath.

"What do you think if we stay here tonight and I cook something for dinner? Then we'll have a cozy evening. There's a great film coming out today that I'd like to see."

"Sure," I agreed.

After the meal we sat on the rather small couch next to each other.

"May I lean on you? Then I can put my feet on the couch. They're getting really cold," she asked me.

"Of course," of course I answered, all gentlemen.

She drew her feet up and swung herself onto the couch so she could lean against my chest and watch the TV. We spread a blanket over us so she wouldn't get even colder.

I smelled the fresh scent of her hair, felt her warmth and her cuddly body.

Again my member began to erect.

I hope she doesn't notice. But I didn't want to change my position either, otherwise she might sit down differently. So it was very pleasant.

Her head was now resting on my shoulder as she watched the film intently. Eventually she put her hand on my stomach. She lay very still. But the warmth seemed to burn a hole in my shirt. After a while she started to move her hand very slowly. She circled over my stomach. Very small circles that slowly grew larger. She came to the edge of my jeans. But only marginally.

Then she took her hand up and put it fully on my jeans, under which my cock was now taut. It felt great. She shifted her position slightly to get a better look. Then she opened my zipper and pulled my pants apart a bit. I didn't wear panties because I enjoyed the feeling of being naked under jeans.

My penis was now almost completely exposed.

She bent down and gently took it in her mouth. She just let my glans slide into her mouth. In between she licked the tip with her tongue.

"Hey, you don't have to do that."

"Fool," she laughed. "I always do what I want to do myself. I think I've fallen in love with you a little bit.

Now shut up and enjoy," she stifled any further protest.

Again she took the tip in her mouth. Very carefully. She did that for quite a while and I really enjoyed it. Then, suddenly, she absorbed him completely. My cock disappeared in her mouth to the root. I groaned. That felt so awesome. Again and again she let it disappear completely in her mouth. Gagged a bit as I thrust against her throat, but that seemed to excite her even more. Spit ran out of her mouth, down my cock onto the sack, which tightened more and more. If she kept this up, it wouldn't be long before I shot my cum down her throat.

"Stop. I'll be right there I want to spoil you too. We still have so much time."

I pulled her chin up and we sank into an intense kiss, letting our tongues dance. In between, I kissed her neck, nibbled her ears and moaned into it because she kept running her hand up and down my penis.

The nibbling and moaning probably turned her on, because her breathing also began to go ragged. Or was it my hand, which I had meanwhile pushed into the pants of her tracksuit from above and which I was stroking over her lace-trimmed panties?

"Do you want to continue watching the movie or shall we cozy up next door?"

“Oh, I know the film inside and out. "It was just an excuse to spend a TV evening with you and get closer to you," she smiled. "It worked out well."

We went next door to my bedroom.

She walked in front of me, briefly pulling down her sweatpants so I could see her tight bottom. Then she snapped the waistband back up. I would do that with today, that incredibly sweet butt!

Once in the bedroom, she fell backwards onto the bed. I wanted to follow her, but she motioned me with a clear hand movement for me to stop.

"Drop your pants. I want to see something too while you can watch me."

I preferred nothing!

I took off my pants and t-shirt.

I stood completely naked against the wall of the room with my cock sticking out stiffly. Natalie slowly unzipped her track jacket, teasingly slowly. Then she pulled both sides back. Her bosom encased in the magical bra was now good for me to see. She squeezed both her mounds together with her arms. How I would like to slide my cock in between or cum on it. Or even better, both!

She reached into the bra with one hand and pulled out a nipple. Slowly she ran her finger over the already hardened bud. Then she pinched her nipple firmly with her index finger and thumb. With a groan, she threw her head back. She seemed to have sensitive breasts.

Then she slipped her other hand into her waistband and played with her crotch. How I would have liked to see more now. My hand was on my cock now, stroking back and forth very slowly.

"But don't cum. I want your juice. Clear?"

I nodded my head in agreement.

Now she stripped her sweatpants down her legs. To do this, she lifted her buttocks slightly. Between her thighs I could see the taut fabric of her panties.

When she pulled her pants over her feet, she let her legs fall wide apart. She pressed firmly with both hands on her mons pubis. A finger seemed to penetrate her vagina through the fabric. She reared up.

With a little yelp, she pulled her panties aside.

Her vagina lay naked in front of me. She was completely shaved around her labia. Only above the clitoris was a small, fire-red hair triangle.

Moaning, she pushed first one, then a second finger into her column. She pushed quickly and watched my tight penis, which I massaged gently.

She looked beautiful!

Only the bra from which one of her wonderful little apples fell out. With her legs spread wide, her fingers thrusting into her hole over and over again.

I couldn't take it anymore and went to the bed to get a closer look at her.

"Well finally! I thought you were going to stay there all night."

She masturbated more and more wildly. Her back arched up while both of her fingers disappeared deep into her vulva.

"Squirt in my face. I want to taste your juice."

I only had to pull my foreskin back twice before my climax was announced. Groaning, the first splash landed on her face and hit her on the forehead. The following ones also landed on her face, which was contorted with lust.

Her orgasm came at the same time. As my cum ran down her face, her body shook in almost spastic motions.

She twitched and reared up again and again.

I was quickly on the bed.

I pushed her panties aside and rammed my penis into her wet vagina. This seemed to prolong her climax.

I thrust into her hard a few times.

Then I collapsed on her, exhausted. She too was flat.

I rolled off her and hugged her. We lay there quietly for a few minutes.

"That was so cool," she whispered in my ear, "I wished for that this morning. Now that the first pressure is gone, we have plenty of time and can enjoy it."

We must have lain like that for a quarter of an hour before my hands wandered about. First I freed her from her bra.

Leaning on my arm, I could look at her now. She was athletically slim. No belly or any love handles, but still very womanly. With a jerk I turned her on her stomach to have a good look at the back as well.

She had an almost small but incredibly sweet ass. But I had already seen that when she came out of the bathroom.

I stroked the shoulder blades, massaging them a bit, which she purred in response.

My hand slowly wandered deeper onto her buttocks. Both hands were now on her buttocks, half in each hand.

I pulled my butt apart very easily.

I could see her small anus. It looked very lovely. Let's see how she reacted. I gently ran a finger through the gap, touched her anus very lightly without staying there. She flinched slightly when I touched her sphincter, but she didn't seem uncomfortable.

I rolled her back onto her back and kissed her breasts. Sucked her warts into my mouth lightly. Biting the tips. Her breathing became a little heavier.

Then I hiked deeper. Licked her belly button with her tongue. Got a little deeper. Wet her dense triangle of pubic hair with my tongue before licking the cheeky protruding clit with the tip of my tongue for the first time.

With a sigh, she pressed my head more firmly onto her sex. I licked her harder. Pulled her pussy lips apart a bit with both hands to thrust her tongue into that pink hole.

I added a finger and thrust it into her vagina. She squirmed more and more under me. Enjoyed this treatment.

I dropped spit from my mouth onto her perineum. With the other hand I stroked the juice in the direction of the rosette, without stopping the treatment of her now sopping wet vagina.

I slowly ran my finger through her buttocks. This time with a little more pressure on her rosette.

"Yes continue. I'll be soon."

Did you mean front or back? Or both?

My finger pressed harder and harder on her anus. Then the resistance was overcome and I slipped into her warm intestines up to the first joint. Not a defensive movement, but rather a push against it.

"More! Fuck me in both holes" she almost screamed.

She could have that!

With two fingers in her vagina and one finger in her gut, I began penetrating her hard and fast.

Then the time came. She came with a violent gasp that made my fingers slip out of her vagina.

She twitched, trembled, and wailed in a way I had never seen a woman do.

She then lay there, breathing heavily.

"Oh, that was so cool. I felt so hard. How do you know I like to be spoiled anally?"

"I didn't know, but thought I'd give it a try," I replied.

"Now I want to feel you. Stick your cock in me."

"Can you do it again?"

"I could always go on. You make me so horny."

I slowly pushed my stiff penis into her vagina. Centimeter by centimetre. I wanted to savor that feeling of first intrusion. I slowly started to push. She was breathing faster again.

Since I had already chummed, we had some time before the juice would shoot up again.

I shagged her for quite a while, while she kept looking into my eyes. She was breathing faster and faster. It was almost a gasp. Then she pushed me away a bit.

"Now fuck my ass."

She turned from under me and got on her knees. As a result, her gorgeous bottom was stretched up. I carefully put the tip of my cock on her rosette, which was still a little open from the previous finger treatment.

I easily pushed the glans through her sphincter. I didn't mean to hurt her. But she had other plans. With a backward jerk, she impaled herself on my spike. Now it was almost completely gone in her intestines.

I slowly started to thrust. Always a little bit deeper, until he had completely disappeared into her.

"Firm. fuck me faster."

I didn't need to be told twice. I pushed harder and harder now. It wouldn't be long before I cummed in this tight hole. Her hand had disappeared between her legs and she was rubbing her clit.

"Squirt it all up my ass," she cheered me on.

Then it was time for me!

I discharged thrust after thrust in her buttocks. Almost at the same time she was ready. She came for the third time that evening. Not as violent as before, but still loudly audible.

"Whoa, now I'm done."

"I hope so," I replied exhaustedly.

"It can still be a nice vacation," she grinned, snuggling up to me, "but now I have to sleep."

She turned to the side and shortly afterwards was already in the realm of dreams.

I looked at this beautiful woman with tenderness.

Was I about to fall in love with her?

Into a Franconia!

That's actually not possible.

But my heart probably decided otherwise.

www.ingramcontent.com/pod-product-compliance
Lightning Source LLC
LaVergne TN
LVHW012058160826
845678LV00014B/2871
* 9 7 9 8 3 5 3 0 0 4 7 7 6 *